AOTCB

Study Guide for the OTR Certification Examination

Editor
Susan McLeod Lang, M.P.H., OTR/L
Director of Examination Development
American Occupational Therapy Certification Board, Inc.

American Occupational Therapy
Certification Board, Inc.
4 Research Place, Suite 160
Rockville, MD 20850-3226

Cover and Interior Design by Cindy Dyer/Dyer Design
Library of Congress Catalogue Number: 94-70543
ISBN 0-9639373-1-6

Printed in the United States of America

Acknowledgements

This study guide would not have been possible without the efforts of the contributors, content reviewers, and student reviewers. These individuals donated their professional expertise and valuable time to ensure that this manual will be helpful for all who use it. The AOTCB staff is thanked for their participation in creating this study guide.

Contributors

Mary M. Arnold, M.A., OTR/L

Ellen DeAustin, OTR

Linda Florey, M.A., OTR, FAOTA

Dairlyn M. Gower, B.A.S., COTA

James P. Klyczek, Ph.D., OTR

Saundra Redding, M.Ed., OTR/L

Pamela Richardson, M.S., OTR/L

Karen M. Romanowski, OTR

Sally Schultz, Ph.D., OTR/L

Dorothy J. Wilson, OTR, FAOTA

Content Reviewers

Program Director Advisory Committee Members

Deborah R. Labovitz, Ph.D., OTR, FAOTA

New York University

Ruth L. Schemm, Ed.D., OTR/L, FAOTA

Thomas Jefferson University

M. Jeanne Madigan, Ed.D., OTR, FAOTA

Virginia Commonwealth University

A special thank you to faculty and students from Towson State University and D'Youville College who reviewed the study guide questions.

Foreword

In response to the many requests for a study guide, the AOTCB is very pleased to offer the *Study Guide for the OTR Certification Examination* as a service to our candidates. Over the past year much time has been spent reviewing the questions and making the content of the study guide representative of the certification examination. The certification examination serves as the final step in preparation to practice as an OTR. The AOTCB is committed to protecting the public by assuring that all certified occupational therapists have completed both an accredited educational program and the required fieldwork and have passed the certification examination. The AOTCB is proud to offer this guide to assist candidates in demonstrating their knowledge on the certification examination.

Elizabeth Cada, M.S., OTR/L, FAOTA
President, AOTCB

Table of Contents

SECTION I Introduction to the Certification Examination

Overview and Purpose of the Study Guide 2

Certification Process

- American Occupational Therapy Certification Board 3
- Certification Examination Development Committee 3
- Job Analysis 3
- Item Development. 3
- Examination Composition 4
- Testing Service 4
- Purpose and History of Certification
  - AOTCB Certification Versus State Regulation 5
- Eligibility Requirements 6

SECTION II Review for the Certification Examination

- Questions Frequently Asked about the Certification Examination 8
- Content Outline 13
- Strategies for Reviewing and Preparing for the Examination 20
- Strategies for Taking the Examination. 21

SECTION III Sample Questions and Answers

- Sample Questions 24
- Answer Key 36
- Questions with Answers and Explanations 38

SECTION IV Selected References

- Selected References 66

Important Note to Examination Candidates and Others

This study guide has been developed in an effort to provide information that may be useful to you in preparing for the AOTCB OTR Certification Examination. This guide does not include all of the material that you should use in preparing for the certification examination. You should use this guide in conjunction with other resources that pertain to the practice of occupational therapy. Enhanced performance on the AOTCB OTR Certification Examination because of or through the use of this book is neither expressed nor implied by the AOTCB, Inc.

This guide is not intended nor suited for use by persons in need of occupational therapy services. If such services are needed, an occupational therapy professional should be consulted.

SECTION I
Introduction to the Certification Examination

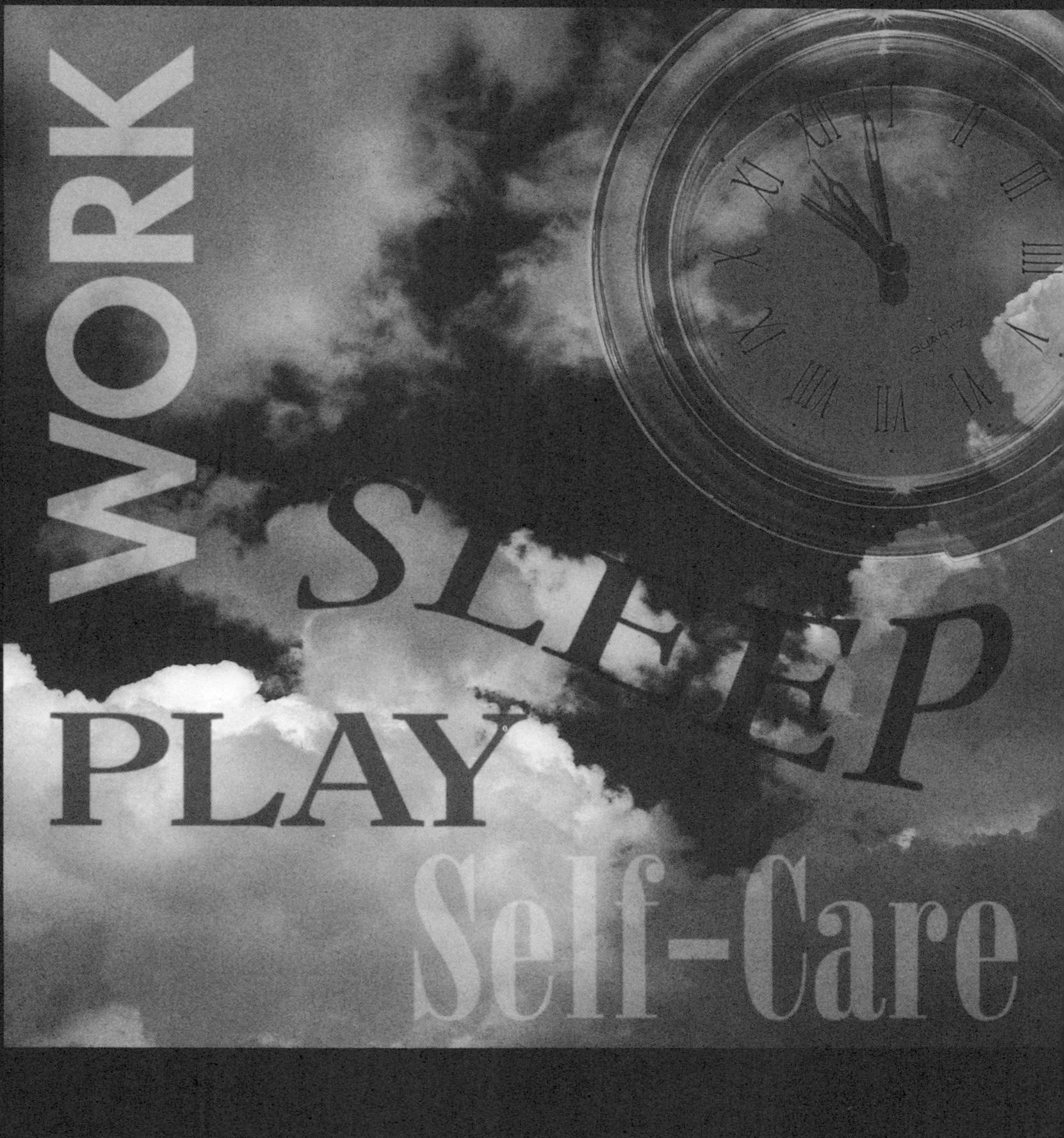

Overview and Purpose of the Study Guide

The study guide is divided into four sections. The first section is an overview of information about how the AOTCB OTR Certification Examination is developed. The second section has the examination specifications, commonly asked questions about the examination, and strategies for taking the examination.

The third section has fifty sample questions in a practice examination format. The AOTCB OTR Certification Examination comprises 200 questions and the examination period is four hours in length; thus, you should be able to complete fifty questions in one hour. Since this study guide contains only fifty sample questions, not all diagnoses or treatment areas will be represented that are on the 200 question examination. The purpose of the study guide questions is not to cover all the material that is covered on the AOTCB OTR Certification Examination but is to illustrate the format of the examination. None of the questions included in this study guide will appear on the AOTCB OTR Certification Examination.

The third section also includes the same fifty questions with explanations for the right and wrong answers. These explanations are designed to facilitate the thought process the candidate should use when answering the questions.

The fourth section is a selected reference list developed from a survey done with OT program directors in 1993. It contains books recommended by the majority of program directors that might be helpful for the candidate to review prior to taking the AOTCB OTR Certification Examination.

This guide should be used as only one tool in preparing for the certification examination. Reviewing your class materials, classroom notes, school textbooks, and fieldwork experiences are important in preparation for the examination. This study guide will supplement your study efforts by giving information on the testing process and the structure of the questions that will be asked on the AOTCB examination.

American Occupational Therapy Certification Board

The American Occupational Therapy Certification Board, Inc. (AOTCB) is responsible for the development and implementation of all policies related to the certification of occupational therapy personnel. The high standards of the certification examinations are ensured by the close working relationship among the AOTCB Certification Examination Development Committee, AOTCB office staff, and test and measurement experts. Most state or jurisdictional regulatory agencies have recognized the use of the AOTCB examinations as a credentialing standard in their jurisdictions.

Certification Examination Development Committee

The examinations are developed by the AOTCB Certification Examination Development Committee (CEDC), a group of content experts (COTAs and OTRs) drawn from a wide variety of work environments and geographical areas. The CEDC is a standing committee of the AOTCB that is composed of fourteen members who serve as content experts for the Occupational Therapist, Registered and Certified Occupational Therapy Assistant certification examinations. The members must have five years experience in their practice area and must be currently spending 40 percent of their time in direct patient care. The members serve a three-year term.

The examination items are written by the CEDC as well as by other COTAs and OTRs who have content expertise and are trained item writers. The item writers are given indepth instruction in writing multiple choice questions by our professional testing agency. All items are reviewed by the CEDC before appearing on the examinations. Item writers use the AOTA *Uniform Terminology for Occupational Therapy*, Second Edition (1989) as a basis for terminology. This publication is available for purchase from the AOTA, 1383 Piccard Drive, Rockville, Maryland 20849-1725, (301) 948-9626.

Job Analysis

The current OTR and COTA certification examinations are based on the results of "*A National Study of the Profession of Occupational Therapy*" completed by the Educational Testing Service in 1991. The study included a survey of approximately 1500 OTR and COTA practitioners and educators. The goal of the survey was to establish the importance of the knowledge of certain tasks for **entry-level** clinicians. The study emphasizes the tasks needed on **entry** into the profession. The content outlines for both examinations were derived from the study and may be found both in the candidate handbook and this study guide.

Item Development

Items which appear on the certification examination have been subjected to rigorous review. Each item has been validated by the CEDC as appropriate for the assessment of the knowledge and skills which are essential and important for entry-level performance as well as important in differentiating adequate from inadequate entry-level performance. The items are also reviewed for bias, making sure that the context, setting, language, descriptions, terminology, and content of the items are inoffensive, free of stereotype, and equally appropriate for all segments of the candidate population, including minority groups.

Examination Composition

The COTA and OTR items are kept in separate item banks and are used only on their respective examinations. Every administration of the examination employs a unique combination of items drawn from the item bank in accordance with the content areas and their associated weightings as identified on the content outlines. The outlines guide the selection of items for each examination and assure that the emphasis on the various content areas and their respective weightings are constant.

Each examination consists of 200 items that use the four-option, multiple choice format. There is only one correct response/answer for each item. All items are equal in weight. No combination answers, such as “All of the Above”, or “A” and “B” are used. Answers are marked on a separate answer sheet. It is to your advantage to **answer every examination item** as all unanswered and incorrect answers carry the same penalty.

Testing Service

The AOTCB contracts with a professional testing company that is responsible for assuring that all of the psychometric principles are followed in test construction and administration activities. The testing company assists the CEDC both in developing the items for the AOTCB examinations and in assuring the content validity and reliability of the AOTCB examination. The testing agency also arranges for the administration of the examination, the scoring of the answer sheets, and the issuing of score reports.

Purpose and History of Certification

AOTCB Certification Versus State Regulation

The AOTCB is a private, nonprofit, nongovernmental agency that administers a national certification program for occupational therapy personnel. Credentials are awarded to persons who have met specific education, fieldwork, and examination requirements. Depending on qualifications, persons may be credentialed as either an Occupational Therapist, Registered (OTR) or as a Certified Occupational Therapy Assistant (COTA).

The purpose of certification, i.e. the awarding of the credentials, is to identify for the public those persons who have demonstrated both the knowledge and the skill necessary to provide occupational therapy services. Thus, the primary purpose of the AOTCB certification program is protection of and service to the public.

The first certification examination for OTRs was administered by the AOTA in 1939 and the first examination for COTAs was given in 1977. In 1986, the AOTCB was created as a new organization, separate from the AOTA. The AOTCB has the sole responsibility for establishing the certification requirements, policies, and procedures for the development and administration of the certification program. The AOTCB Board of Directors consists of OTRs, COTAs, and public directors.

At the present time, AOTCB certification continues for a person's lifetime unless it is removed by a disciplinary action. There is no fee to maintain this certification. As of 1994, forty-nine states plus the District of Columbia and Puerto Rico have some form of regulation for the profession of occupational therapy. The form of state regulation includes trademark laws, registration, certification, and licensure. It is important to realize that AOTCB certification is separate from state regulation, which requires a separate application process. The majority of these jurisdictions recognize certification from AOTCB as one of the requirements for state or jurisdictional credentialing. This credentialing ensures minimum entry-level standards for safe practice as an OTR or COTA.

Eligibility Requirements

The eligibility requirements for admission to the certification examination for Occupational Therapist, Registered (OTR) are as follows:

1. For entry-level U.S. graduates of baccalaureate, post-baccalaureate certificate, and master's degree programs for occupational therapists:
   - The candidate must be a **GRADUATE** of an occupational therapy education program accredited by the Accreditation Council for OT Education.
   - The candidate must have successfully completed the therapist-level fieldwork and must have met all of the requirements for graduation by the day before the examination is to be administered. It is not necessary to have completed the graduation exercises.
   - The program director must verify the completion of all academic and fieldwork requirements and notify the AOTCB of the candidate's eligibility to take the examination. **The submission of inaccurate or misleading information concerning the completion of the requirements for certification will prohibit the candidate's taking the examination and/or could result in the censure, suspension, or revocation of certification of the candidate.**

2. For Foreign Graduates:
   - Foreign candidates must have successfully completed all the academic and fieldwork requirements of an approved occupational therapy program.
   - The candidate's *"Application to Determine Eligibility to Take the Certification Examination"* for OTR must be approved by the AOTCB.

Please note: Candidates for whom English is a second language may not use a dictionary and are not permitted to have extra time due to language difficulty. Candidates are advised to prepare by studying English if there is a concern about understanding the test questions due to language difficulties.

It should be noted that each exam candidate has to sign the following pledge. On the cover of each examination booklet, you will find the following statement:

By taking this examination I hereby acknowledge that I understand the following:

(1) That this examination is the exclusive property of the American Occupational Therapy Certification Board.

(2) That this examination and the items contained therein are protected by federal copyright law. No part of this examination may be copied, reproduced in part or whole by any means whatsoever, including memorization, unless previously authorized by the American Occupational Therapy Certification Board.

(3) That theft or attempted theft of an examination booklet or any of its pages is punishable as a felony.

(4) That my participation in any irregularity occurring during this examination, such as giving or obtaining unauthorized information or aid, as evidenced by observation or subsequent statistical analysis may be sufficient cause to terminate my participation, invalidate the results of my examination and/or take other appropriate action.

SECTION II
Review for the the Certification Examination

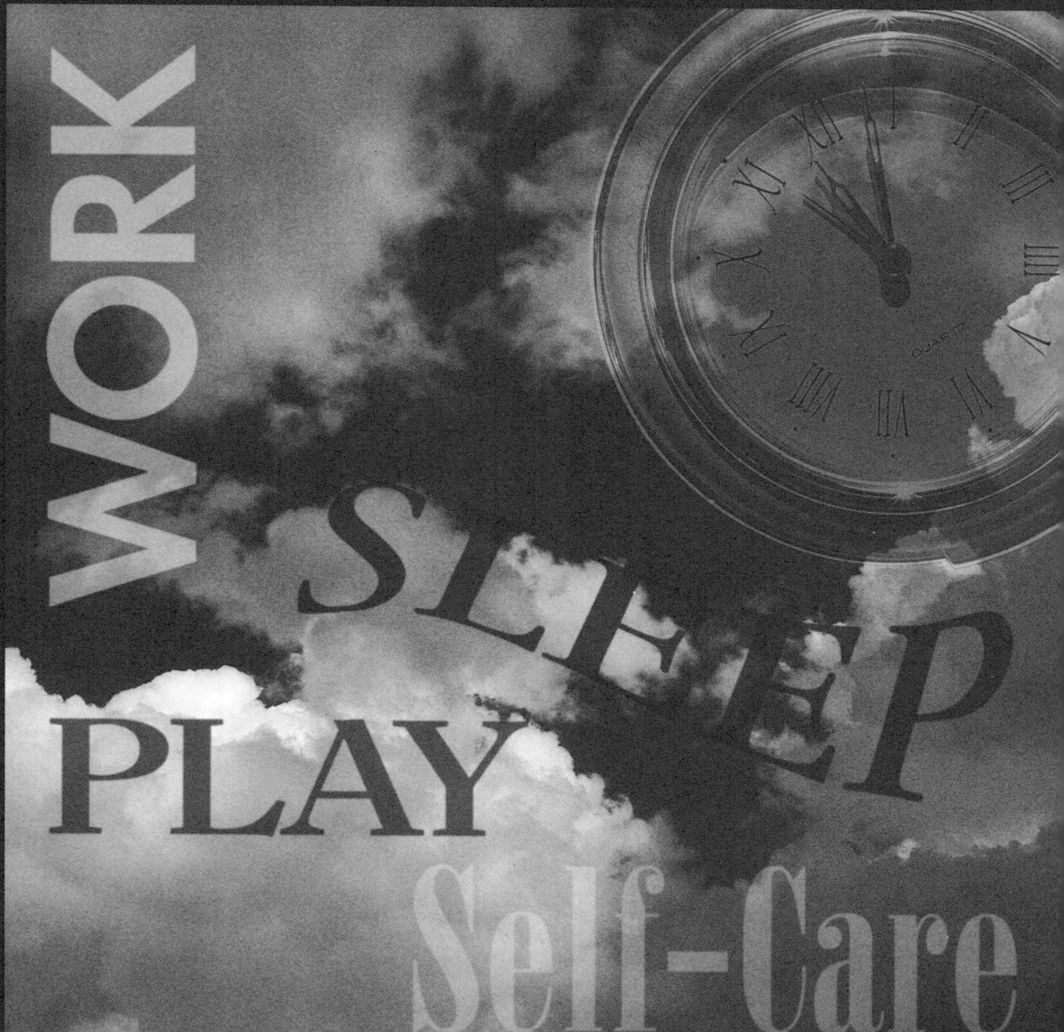

Questions Frequently Asked about the Certification Examination

1. **How do I apply to take the examination?**
When you become eligible to take the examination the program director at your school will submit your name and address to the AOTCB as being eligible to sit for the certification examination. The AOTCB will send you the "Candidate Handbook" with an application to be completed and returned to the testing service. Candidate handbooks are sent in September for the January examination and in March for the July examination.

2. **What is the average reading level of the certification examination?**
The average reading level required for the OTR examination is at the second year of college.

3. **What standard abbreviations may be used?**
Only standard abbreviations and acronyms are used on the certification examinations. They include, but are not limited to, the following:

ADL	Activities of Daily Living
AIDS	Acquired Immune Deficiency Syndrome
COTA	Certified Occupational Therapy Assistant
CVA	Cerebral Vascular Accident
DIP	Distal Interphalangeal
OT	Occupational Therapy
OTR	Occupational Therapist, Registered
PIP	Proximal Interphalangeal
POMR	Problem-Oriented Medical Record
ROM	Range of Motion
SOAP	Subjective, Objective, Assessment, and Plan

The use of the term "frame of reference" on the examination refers to models, paradigms, and theories.

4. **How long is the examination?**
The examination consists of 200 multiple choice questions.

5. **How much time will I have to take the examination?**
Candidates have four hours to take the examination.

6. **How will I provide my answers?**
At the test site, candidates will be provided with a separate answer sheet with a series of circles that you will fill in with a #2 pencil to record answers. Please be sure to provide only **one** answer per item. All answer sheets are machine scored. Completely fill in the space in which you are recording your answer and carefully erase all stray marks, as these could be scored as unintended answers. A sample answer sheet has been provided in this booklet for your use in taking the practice

test. During the AOTCB examination, answers recorded in the test booklet but not on the answer sheet will not be scored.

7. **How is the examination scored?**
Following the administration of each examination, members of the Certification Examination Development Committee (CEDC) and measurement experts from the testing service evaluate the statistical properties of each item of the examination. When candidates do not perform on a particular item as expected, that item is closely evaluated to determine whether it is flawed in any way. If the content experts agree that an item is flawed, then appropriate adjustments to the scoring are made. One adjustment can be that all candidates receive credit for any item that is flawed.

Every form of the certification examination employs a unique combination of items. No two forms are identical from one administration to the next. While each administration of the AOTCB examination is designed to fairly assess the knowledge and skills required for entry-level practice, it is to be expected that there will be a slight fluctuation in the overall level of difficulty from one administration of the examination to another. Such disparities are minor and should not be of concern to the candidates because the passing score for each form is statistically adjusted to compensate for any fluctuations in difficulty level from one administration to another.

The procedure, which is referred to as equating, ensures that candidates of comparable proficiency will be equally likely to pass the examination regardless of fluctuations in the overall difficulty level of the examination from one administration to another. Thus, no candidate will suffer any unintentional penalty due to having taken a form of the examination that turns out to be somewhat more difficult than other forms. Conversely, no advantage will be gained by any candidate who happens to take a form of the examination that is less difficult than other forms. Therefore from the point of view of examination difficulty, candidates have an equal and fair opportunity to achieve a passing score on the examination at each administration.

Along with the equating process, statistical procedures are used to convert raw scores (number correct) to "scaled scores" that are equivalent for all administrations of the examination. The scaled score is not a "number correct" or "percent correct" score. Your results will be reported as a scaled score, on a scale ranging from 300 to 600 points. You must obtain a scaled score of at least 450 in order to pass the examination.

8. **Is the examination criterion-referenced or norm-referenced?**
The certification examination is a criterion-referenced examination. The scoring of the examination may be different from many of the examinations you took while in school. Those examinations were quite often norm-referenced, meaning that your performance on the examination was compared with that of others taking the examination. When norm-referenced examinations are "graded on a bell curve," the test score is adjusted to take into consideration the performance of others taking the

examination. If the highest possible score on the examination is 100 points and the highest score achieved is 85, then the score of 85 points becomes the top score or "A" and all other scores are adjusted accordingly.

In contrast, on a criterion-referenced examination your performance is not compared with others taking the examination. On the AOTCB certification examination, you must obtain a score equal to or higher than the "passing score" in order to pass. The passing score represents an absolute standard and does not depend on the performance of other candidates taking this administration of the examination. The minimum passing score on the examination was set by content experts using the modified-Angoff with data standard-setting methodology. To pass the examination, you must obtain a minimum scaled score of 450. This passing score remains unchanged from one administration to another. The equating process will adjust for any changes in the level of difficulty from one administration of the examination to another.

9. **How does the AOTCB comply with Americans with Disabilities Act and provide special accommodations?**
A candidate with a documented disability (including a visual, orthopedic, or hearing impairment; health impairment; or learning, emotional, or multiple disabilities) who needs modification of the usual testing conditions may request special testing accommodations (e.g., one hour extra time or a reader) to take the certification examination on regularly scheduled national test dates. The candidate should refer to the "AOTCB Candidate Handbook" for the specific process used to request special accommodations.

10. **What if I do not pass the examination?**
If you do not pass the examination, you have the opportunity to retake the examination. You must retake the entire examination and pay the full application fee again. You will be sent another candidate handbook and application for the next administration of the examination. You must notify the AOTCB of any change of address, so that you can receive this information. Information about the application process for the next administration is provided on your score report. If you do not register to take the next scheduled administration of the examination, you will no longer be sent the Candidate Handbook and application for any future administrations. You will have to contact the AOTCB to request a Candidate Handbook and application if you do not sit for the next administration of the examination.

If you do not pass the examination, you may wish to contact the regulatory board in the state/jurisdiction in which you are presently working in order to determine whether you are still able to practice.

You may wish to contact your program director to determine whether he or she can be of any assistance to you in your further preparation for the examination. Scores identified by name are not reported to your program director or school so they will not know whether a candidate has or has not passed the examination.

This is an example of a score report that is sent to candidates that do not pass the examination. **Passing candidates are sent the score that they received on the examination only.**

AMERICAN OCCUPATIONAL THERAPY CERTIFICATION BOARD, INC.
Results on the Occupational Therapist, Registered (OTR) Examination
Tested January 22, 1994

Your score on the examination is 398.
REGRETFULLY, YOU HAVE NOT PASSED THE EXAMINATION.

Content Area	Passing Score	% of Exam in this area	Your Score
TOTAL TEST SCORE	450	100.0%	398
Assess Occupational Performance		15.0%	366
Develop Treatment Plan		24.0%	359
Implement Treatment Plan		20.0%	374
Evaluate Treatment Plan		09.0%	439
Develop Discharge Plan		07.5.%	503
Org. and Manage Services		12.5%	455
Promote Professional Practice		11.5%	395

A TOTAL TEST SCORE of 450 or higher is required to pass. The lowest possible Score is 300 and the highest possible score is 600.

KEEP A COPY OF THIS DOCUMENT FOR YOUR FILES

Above is a report of your performance on the Occupational Therapist, Registered (OTR) Examination. Your scores on the test are reported as converted scores. The number of items you answered correctly has been transformed arithmetically to a scale score. The subscores for major content areas are provided for diagnostic purposes only. They cannot be used to determine a final score or a passing score. If any of your subscores are below 450, then you are advised to focus your study on these areas as you review.

11. **Is there a limit on the number of times that I can take the examination?**
The AOTCB places no limits on the number of times you may take the certification examination. If you are taking the examination for licensure purposes you are advised to contact the regulatory board for information regarding the number of times you are permitted to take the examination and still be eligible for licensure in that state.

12. **Are there questions about AOTA on the examination?**
No, the American Occupational Therapy Association is a professional membership organization and testing of information about this organization is not essential for entry-level practice of the OTR or COTA.

13. **Are the questions on the COTA and OTR examinations the same?**
No, all questions on the two certification examinations are different.

Content Outline

The examination content outline has been developed to identify the major and specific work activities that define the entry-level practice of OTRs along with the knowledge required to perform those activities. This outline is organized as follows:

- The first statement, identified by a roman numeral, represents the domain. A domain is the principal area of responsibility or activity comprising the job of an OTR.
- The next statement, identified by a small letter "a", "b", etc., is referred to as the task statement. A task statement is defined as a specific, goal-directed set of activities having a common objective or type of output. These statements serve to further delineate the domain.
- Each group of task statements is followed by a list of knowledge statements. These statements represent the knowledge required to perform the tasks which precede them. Each knowledge statement can apply to several of the task statements under which it is listed. For example, in the OTR outline under Domain I, the knowledge statement 'Observation techniques' could be required for adequate performance of any task listed under Domain I, from "a" through "e."
- The general knowledge statements found at the end of the content outline reflect knowledge required to perform tasks which are found in one or more of the content domains. These statements represent general knowledge which forms a foundation for the practice of occupational therapy and therefore can be linked with several content domains and many task statements. The general knowledge statements are useful for giving the candidate an understanding of basic and fundamental knowledge needed in entry-level occupational therapy practice.

Preparation for the AOTCB examination should be focused on all elements of the content outline. Items on the examination are distributed across the major practice areas and diagnoses in occupational therapy.

Examination Content Outline
Occupational Therapist Registered (OTR)

Approximate % of Questions:
The percentage may vary slightly from examination to examination.

15% **I. Assess Individual's Occupational Performance**

a. Obtain and review pertinent background information
b. Plan and select screening and evaluation methods and tools
c. Interview individual and/or significant others
d. Observe individual's performance
e. Formulate clinical hypotheses
f. Administer appropriate evaluations for assessment
g. Analyze assessment information
h. Develop recommendations for referral to other service(s) if needed
i. Document assessment results using appropriate terminology
j. Integrate theoretical knowledge base(s) into assessment

Assessment–Knowledge Statements

Observation techniques
Information sources (e.g., persons, records, charts, forms)
Interviewing techniques
Individual differences (e.g., sociocultural, age, gender)
Characteristics of standardized and nonstandardized assessments
Assessment instruments used in OT practice and what they measure
Factors to consider in selection of assessment instruments
Test administration procedures
Test interpretation
Use of activities for assessment

23% **II. Develop Treatment Plan**

a. Communicate with individual to establish goals
b. Collaborate in setting goals and planning treatment
c. Document/report involvement of individual in goal setting
d. Develop and document measurable long-term goals
e. Develop sequential, measurable short-term goals
f. Analyze activities to facilitate goal achievement
g. Select specific treatment activities consistent with goals
h. Grade treatment activities to facilitate goal achievement
i. Select specific treatment modalities, techniques, and environment
j. Select tools, equipment, materials, and location needed
k. Adapt techniques, equipment, and materials
l. Estimate frequency and duration of treatment
m. Consider daily regimen of individual in scheduling treatment

n. Document treatment plan
o. Integrate theoretical knowledge base(s) into treatment planning

Treatment Planning–Knowledge Statements

Role and function of other service providers
Role and function of treatment teams
Health risks to the individual related to disability or disease
Goal-setting
Tools, equipment, and materials commonly used in OT practice
Media, methods, and modalities commonly used on OT practice
Components of a treatment plan
Activities grading
Ways to identify community resources

19% **III. Implement Treatment Plan**

a. Explain plan to individual, significant others, service providers
b. Use OT activities and methods to achieve treatment goals
c. Physically manage the individual (e.g., positioning)
d. Instruct individual in functional mobility (e.g., transfer)
e. Select and provide assistive/adaptive/orthotic devices
f. Design and construct assistive/adaptive/orthotic devices
g. Instruct individual in care and use of assistive adaptive/orthotic devices
h. Evaluate effectiveness of assistive/adaptive/orthotic devices
i. Instruct individual regarding preventive strategies
j. Take precautions related to contraindications and safety of others
k. Instruct individual about potential health risks
l. Prepare a home program for the individual and/or significant others
m. Integrate theoretical knowledge base(s) into implementation

Treatment Implementation–Knowledge Statements

Types and functions of assistive devices and adaptive equipment
Types and functions of orthotic devices
Design and fabrication of adaptive equipment and assistive devices
Design and fabrication of orthotic devices
Technologies used in OT interventions
Behavior management techniques
Stress management techniques
Instructional methods
ADL activities
Work activities
Play/leisure activities
Arts and crafts
Work hardening
Positioning and handling techniques
Transfer techniques
Functional mobility techniques

Compensatory techniques
Work simplification techniques
Cognitive levels and impact on performance
Group process and dynamics
Time management strategies
Social skills training
Verbal and nonverbal communication techniques
Sensory integration techniques
Sensory stimulation techniques
Perceptual motor activities
Motor planning activities
Techniques for facilitating and inhibiting muscle tone
Reflex inhibition techniques
Techniques for facilitating oral-motor control
Techniques for facilitating fine-motor coordination/dexterity
Activities to improve or maintain strength
Activities to improve or maintain endurance
Activities to improve or maintain range of motion

10% **IV. Evaluate Treatment Plan**

a. Reassess and document individual's functional performance
b. Discuss progress with individual, significant others, etc.
c. Identify need for change in treatment plan
d. Modify treatment plan
e. Document changes in treatment plan
f. Integrate theoretical knowledge base(s) into evaluation

9% **V. Develop Discharge Plan**

a. Determine individual's need for OT services after discharge
b. Identify community resources
c. Develop discharge plan
d. Discuss discharge plan with individual, significant others, etc.
e. Recommend environmental adaptations and resources
f. Write discharge summary

Evaluation and Discharge–Knowledge Statements (These knowledge statements apply to content listed under sections IV and V above.)
Expected outcomes of various treatments
Responses to unexpected reactions during treatment
Environmental barriers and adaptations/modification
Psychological and social barriers and methods for change
Discharge planning process

12% **VI. Organize and Manage Services**

a. Respond to a request or referral for OT services
b. Document a response to a request or referral for OT services
c. Assure compliance with organization policies
d. Promote OT services to relevant individuals
e. Adhere to standards for safe and efficient operation
f. Report and document all accidents and incidents
g. Comply with agency or program accreditation requirements
h. Maintain supplies and equipment
i. Participate in quality assurance program/program evaluation

Organization and Management of Services–Knowledge Statements

Referral process
Health and safety standards (e.g., universal infection control)
Emergency and safety procedures
Environmental hazards in the OT setting
Reimbursement for OT services
Purpose of quality assurance and program evaluation
Purpose of organizational policies and procedures
Maintenance of equipment and supplies

12% **VII. Promote Professional Practice**

a. Explain roles, functions, and benefits of OT services to the public
b. Comply with professional codes of ethics
c. Comply with occupational therapy standards of practice
d. Comply with state regulations governing occupational therapy
e. Report unethical, illegal, or unsafe practices
f. Secure adequate malpractice and liability coverage when applicable
g. Update knowledge of theories and techniques in OT

Professional Practice–Knowledge Statements

Patient's rights (e.g., confidentiality, right to refuse treatment)
Occupational therapy codes of ethics
Occupational therapy standards of practice
Credentialing process and requirements of OT personnel
Legal liability related to OT services
Changes and trends in OT practice

General Knowledge Statements

Biological sciences
Physical sciences
Behavioral sciences
Medical terminology
Diagnostically related contradictions and precautions
Clinical reasoning process

Human Development and Function

Physical development
Deficits in physical functioning
Cognitive development
Deficits in cognitive functioning
Psychosocial development
Deficits in psychosocial functioning
Sensorimotor development
Deficits in sensorimotor functioning

General Occupational Therapy

Theories
Information resources
Treatment principles and approaches
Principles of group design
Activity analysis
Terminology
General indicators for OT intervention

Occupational Performance Areas

ADL
Work
Play or leisure

Sensorimotor Performance Components

Sensory awareness
Sensory processing (e.g., tactile, proprioceptive)
Perceptual skills
Reflexes
Range of motion
Muscle tone
Strength
Endurance
Postural control
Soft tissue integrity
Activity tolerance

Gross-motor coordination
Crossing the midline
Laterality
Bilateral integration
Praxis
Fine-motor coordination/dexterity
Visual-motor integration
Oral-motor control

Cognitive Integration and Cognitive Components

Level of arousal
Orientation
Recognition
Attention span
Memory (e.g., short term, long term, remote, recent)
Sequencing
Spatial relations
Problem solving/decision making
Generalizations of learning

Psychosocial Skills and Psychological Components

Roles
Values
Interests
Initiation of activity
Termination of activity
Self-concept
Self-control
Verbal and nonverbal communication
Self-expression
Coping skills
Time management

Documentation

Formats (e.g., SOAP, POMR, narrative)
Content related to steps in treatment process

Strategies for Reviewing and Preparing for the Examination

Materials to Review

The certification examination is a rigorous examination. You are advised to prepare a plan of study which allows for several months of review. In preparation for the examination, it is recommended that candidates review class notes, texts, and journals in occupational therapy using the content outlines as a guide to preparation for the examination.

You may wish to organize your study materials in accordance with the major headings identified on the content outline and organize your study time and emphasis in proportion to the weight given the content area on the examination.

Methods of Study

A candidate must select his or her best method of study. This may be auditory with someone asking questions or visual with practice tests and reviewing notes. Some persons find it helpful to study in groups. The advantages to group study can be a sharing of information from different fieldwork settings and discussion of various content areas.

The examination is practice based which means you are expected to apply your clinical knowledge in clinical scenarios.

You may wish to develop a calendar of study that includes content, day, and time. This breaks the process of studying down into a manageable size and prevents feeling overwhelmed when needing to study such a large number of content areas.

Techniques for Review

1. Review materials in blocks by content area. This might include content areas from the test outline such as assessing occupational performance, developing treatment plan, etc. Think about the materials that you have reviewed and then summarize this for yourself and take a break.
2. Develop your own outline of your strengths and weaknesses in relation to the content areas. This outline will be your self-assessment and will highlight the areas where you need more study and those areas that you have mastered. For example, this outline might include
   1) Need intensive study
   2) Need to study
   3) Adequate knowledge, but should review
   4) Strong area, no additional study needed.

   This type of an assessment would allow you to prioritize the various areas that you need to study.
3. Write out notes as you review various study materials. Summarize the key points and relate them to the test outline.

4. Think about patients or clients studied in your educational program and patients or clients you treated during your fieldwork where the particular content that you are studying could be applied. Analyze these cases in regard to the knowledge you needed to perform the occupational therapy intervention. For example, determine the knowledge you needed regarding the structure and function of the human body, developmental levels, environmental factors, occupational theory, assessments, evaluations, and techniques and procedures for interventions. Performing this analysis makes the knowledge that you are studying more relevant and important to you as a future OTR. Material that is viewed to be relevant and important enhances one's ability to retain information.

5. Plan to overstudy for the examination by beginning your study early and regularly reviewing areas that you have studied in the past. Repetition is a valuable tool in retaining information.

Strategies for Taking the Examination

Dealing With Test Anxiety

This is a high-stakes examination and some apprehension would be normal. The major way to cope with normal test anxiety is with the proper study before the examination and the right attitude in taking the examination. Attitudes are thought to be learned; therefore, a new attitude toward testing can be learned. It may be helpful to visualize yourself being successful in the test situation. The background for this type of visualization can be based on the educational preparation, fieldwork, and life experience that you will be taking with you into the examination. Also, some candidates find relaxation techniques helpful in reducing overall anxiety. Acknowledging and developing a strategy to deal with test anxiety can help prepare the candidate before entering the testing situation.

Preparations Before the Examination

- You may want to obtain a map to the test site.
- Also if the test site is in an unfamiliar area, you may want to make a trip there to check your route.
- The candidate that is taking the test out of town may want to arrive in the city of the test site one day early.
- Get plenty of sleep the night before.
- Keep all of your physical routines the same. Eat a similar breakfast to the one that you eat most mornings.
- Wear comfortable clothes.
- Make sure to check the weather report to allow for extra travel time if needed.
- Arrive at the test site early so that you have time to relax and calm yourself.
- It might be helpful not to talk much with other candidates who are very anxious. This may increase your own anxiety.
- Bring several #2 pencils, eraser, watch, admission ticket, and a means of photo identification to the test site.

Being Test Wise

Being test wise means having the ability to take cues from the test situation that allow you to obtain a score that is appropriate for your level of knowledge of the subject being tested.

1. Pay attention to the directions given by the proctor and those that are printed in the test booklet.
2. Read each stem (first part of the question) carefully and think about the possible right answer before looking at the four options.
3. Look at each option and try to eliminate wrong choices and then select the best answer from the remaining choices.
4. There is no penalty for guessing. Be sure to answer all questions.
5. Answer those questions that you are sure of first and then come back to answer those questions that you have initially left unanswered. This is an effective strategy because each question counts the same amount toward your total score. You will need to be careful to skip a space on your machine scored sheet. You may also wish to mark unanswered questions in your test booklet. This technique gives you more opportunities for success because when you return to the difficult questions you are not as pressed for time.
6. Pacing yourself is very important. You have four hours to take a 200-item examination so keep track of your time and allow about one minute and 12 seconds per question.
7. There are no trick questions.
8. Be sure to pay attention to qualifiers or key words such as NOT, LEAST, FIRST, BEST, ONLY, EXCEPT. These words can definitely have a strong impact on the interpretation of the item.
9. Do not read more into the question than is stated in the question. Pay attention to the information contained in the question.

Best wishes for your success on the examination!

References

If candidates need more information or assistance with skills in test taking, they should contact the learning resources or guidance counselors at their university or college.

Feder, B. 1979. *The Complete Guide to Taking Tests*. Prentice Hall, Inc., Englewood Cliffs, N.J.

Fluitt, J. and C. Gifford. 1988. *Test Taking Made Easier*. The Interstate Printers and Publishers, Inc. Danville, Ill.

Woodley, K. 1978. *Test Wiseness Test Taking Skills for Adults*. Second Edition, McGraw-Hill, New York, N.Y.

SECTION III
Sample Questions & Answers

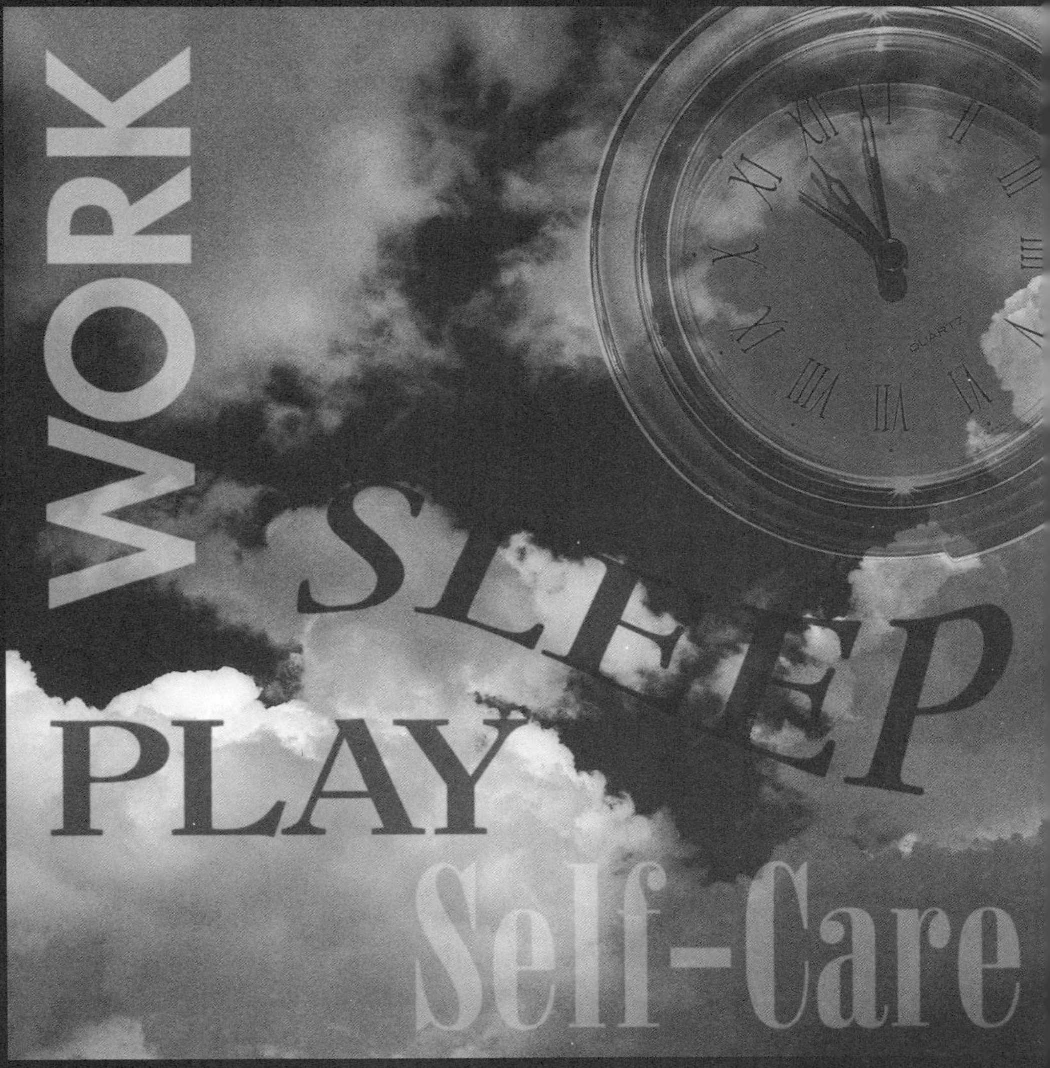

Reminder: Success on the 50 sample questions does not guarantee success on the 200-item AOTCB certification examination.

DIRECTIONS

It is recommended that you use the practice test in a one-hour time frame to estimate your ability to pace yourself while taking the AOTCB examination. During the one-hour practice test period, you will have approximately one to two minutes per question. A sample answer sheet has been provided to practice completing the same type of machine scored answer sheet that is used in the AOTCB examination.

1. A child with fetal alcohol syndrome may display any of the following **EXCEPT**:

   A. speech delays.
   B. macrocephaly.
   C. behavior problems.
   D. average intelligence scores.

2. Which of the following is the **BEST** example of the application of the behavioral frame of reference to facilitate learning?

   A. Discussion to develop insight into the consequences of past actions.
   B. Problem solving to determine the most effective means of performing a task.
   C. Praise to reinforce appropriate social interaction.
   D. Repetition and drill to memorize a sequence of steps for performing a task.

3. Which of the following deficits may be present as a result of a peripheral nerve injury?

   A. Spasticity, decreased muscle strength, and decreased active ROM.
   B. Decreased passive ROM, impaired sensation, and tremor.
   C. Decreased active ROM, decreased muscle tone, and impaired coordination.
   D. Impaired motor planning, decreased muscle strength, and decreased active ROM.

4. An OTR observes another OTR using an incorrect technique to complete a stand pivot transfer with a patient. The OTR who observes the improper transfer has a responsibility to:

   A. report the matter to the OT supervisor immediately.
   B. report it to the OT supervisor if it happens again.
   C. instruct the therapist in the proper technique with the patient present.
   D. talk with the therapist in private about proper stand pivot transfer technique.

5. A realistic functional goal for a patient with complete C_4 quadriplegia would be:

   A. operation of a computer using a head switch.
   B. independence in sliding board transfer.
   C. independence in upper-extremity dressing.
   D. self-feeding with wrist support and adaptive utensils.

6. Which of the following approaches is **LEAST** threatening to an adolescent with schizophrenia who is withdrawn and apprehensive?

   A. Allowing permissiveness.
   B. Providing close supervision.
   C. Providing a variety of activities.
   D. Establishing a set schedule.

7. An OTR is performing a motor assessment on a child with cerebral palsy. When the child turns his head to look at an object placed in his hand, his arm extends and he drops the object. The OTR suspects that this is due to:

   A. poorly coordinated visual pursuits.
   B. asymmetrical tonic neck reflex.
   C. poorly integrated grasp reflex.
   D. upper extremity spasticity.

8. A patient unable to "blow" on command can spontaneously blow out a match placed in front of the face. This is an example of which of the following deficits?

   A. Agnosia.
   B. Ideomotor apraxia.
   C. Ataxia.
   D. Constructional apraxia.

9. The Medicare program was designed **PRIMARILY** to provide medical coverage for:

   A. low-income persons.
   B. people aged 65 and over.
   C. retired persons.
   D. people who have been disabled 12 months or more.

10. Which of the following would be **MOST** difficult for a child with motor planning problems to perform on a scooter board?

    A. Sitting on the scooter board and pulling self along a taut rope with hand-over-hand motion.
    B. Maintaining prone position while being pushed through an obstacle course.
    C. Maintaining balance on the scooter board while being pulled by the OTR.
    D. Going down a ramp in prone position with legs extended.

11. Which of the following statements is an example of objective data when writing a SOAP note?

    A. The patient has 30 degrees of elbow flexion.
    B. The patient will be able to achieve 50 degrees of elbow flexion.
    C. The patient is unable to comb hair due to arm pain.
    D. "I cannot move my right arm without it hurting."

12. An OTR employed in a public school is asked to give a presentation to parents and staff regarding the role of OT in a special education program. Which of the following would be **MOST** effective in presenting the scope of educationally related OT services to this audience?

    A. A description of the types of assessments used to identify students in need of OT services.
    B. A demonstration of equipment most frequently used by school-based OTRs.
    C. A simulation of a therapy session with a child from the OTR's caseload.
    D. A discussion of problems typically addressed by school-based OTRs and service delivery options.

13. An OTR observes that a patient with a spinal cord injury has an improperly fitting wheelchair. The **MOST IMMEDIATE** safety concern of the OTR would be the patient's:

    A. skin integrity.
    B. development of scoliosis.
    C. being unable to propel the wheelchair.
    D. being uncomfortable because of the height of the armrests.

14. A patient is working on a copper tooling project and cuts his finger. The OTR should **FIRST:**

    A practice universal precautions and apply direct pressure to the wound.
    B. contact the physician before initiating any treatment.
    C. document the incident and have the patient return to his room.
    D. report the injury to the patient's nurse.

15. How should paints and paint thinners be stored in an OT clinic?

    A. In a well-ventilated closed metal cabinet.
    B. On shelves in a locked storeroom.
    C. In a well-ventilated closed wooden cabinet.
    D. On open shelves in the craft area.

16. A 16-year-old adolescent who has a cognitive disability and an adjustment disorder, not otherwise specified, is being discharged to his family home from an acute care psychiatric setting. In planning for discharge, the **FIRST** activity for the OTR to consider would be:

    A. planning an appropriate home program.
    B. providing aftercare recommendations and referrals.
    C. educating the family and the patient for transition to community.
    D. evaluating the patient's home environment.

17. An OTR receives a referral for a 12-month-old with spastic quadriplegic cerebral palsy. In addition to an assessment of motor development, which of the following types of evaluations are **MOST** appropriate in an initial assessment?

    A. Reflex testing and feeding evaluation.
    B. Reflex testing and sensory evaluation.
    C. Visual perception evaluation and ADL evaluation.
    D. Sensory evaluation and ADL evaluation.

QUESTIONS 18 AND 19 REFER TO THE FOLLOWING INFORMATION:

An 18-year-old female was hospitalized because she was unable to concentrate and unable to sleep. On admission, her speech was rapid, she was hyperactive, and she began organizing patients' activities for the evening. She became interested in several projects after entering OT.

18. Which of the following would be the **MOST APPROPRIATE** goal for this patient?

    A. Improve work skills.
    B. Increase self-control.
    C. Increase frustration tolerance.
    D. Increase problem-solving ability.

SEE INFORMATION PRECEDING QUESTION 18

19. Which of the following would be the **MOST APPROPRIATE** activity for this patient to achieve the initial goal?

   A. Sketching.
   B. Tile project.
   C. Menu planning.
   D. Leather carving.

20. A patient with a spinal cord injury has difficulty dealing with anger about his limitations. Which of the following actions is an example of **projection** used as a defense mechanism?

   A. The patient tells the OTR that "50% of the nurses on the unit should be doing something else for a living. They think we're second class citizens just because we're in wheelchairs."
   B. During training in electric wheelchair skills, the patient frequently comments, "I can't wait to start riding my motorcycle again!"
   C. The patient tells the other patients that he is going to get his hair cut just like his therapist's and buy the same type of clothes as his therapist's.
   D. The patient states "I am going to get much better seats at the ball game now that I am in a wheelchair."

21. Which of the following OT treatments is **NOT** recommended for patients with degenerative diseases of the central nervous system?

   A. Instruction in energy conservation and work simplification techniques.
   B. Establishment of an aggressive, resistive exercise program.
   C. Provision of assistive devices.
   D. Recommendation of workplace modifications.

22. An 82-year-old who lives alone is forgetful, confused, and disoriented to time. Which of the following approaches would be **MOST** appropriate in assessing the self-care skills of this patient?

   A. Interview the family regarding the patient's self-care skills.
   B. Ask the patient to describe self-care routine.
   C. Observe the patient's performance of self-care routine.
   D. Interview the family regarding environmental safety hazards in patient's home.

23. The length of time a child is able to attend to a task is most directly related to:

   A. memory.
   B. previous experience.
   C. developmental age.
   D. role expectations.

24. A 20-year-old patient hospitalized with a diagnosis of schizophrenia begins to hear voices and walks to the staircase to peer over. The patient says, "I want to kill the voices." The **MOST APPROPRIATE** response for the OTR would be to:

A. ask the patient to identify the voices.
B. talk to the patient while moving the patient from the staircase.
C. discuss the voices and why the patient wants to kill them.
D. tell the patient that the voices are not really there.

25. Which of the following is the primary role of the OTR during the initial phase of cardiac rehabilitation?

A. Assessment of vital signs during simulated work task evaluation.
B. Assessment of cardiovascular responses to sustained standing.
C. Initiation of a progressive upper extremity exercise program.
D. Identification of ways to decrease energy expenditure during self-care tasks.

26. Which of the following would be a long-term goal for an adult with a sudden onset of blindness?

A. Independent coin identification and check writing.
B. Independent bathing, grooming, and dressing.
C. Independent living and exploration of employment options.
D. Independent time-telling and schedule management.

27. Mobile arm supports would help a person with proximal upper extremity weakness perform all of the following activities **EXCEPT:**

A. upper body dressing.
B. self-feeding.
C. participation in tabletop board games.
D. operation of an electric wheelchair.

28. Which of the following activities would be **BEST** for assessing a patient's organizational and planning skills?

A. Adding up the total coupon savings from a grocery bill.
B. Preparing a grocery list for bag lunches for a group lunch.
C. Studying home safety and listing the steps to put out a fire.
D. Identifying the times for three programs using a TV schedule.

29. A child with constructional dyspraxia will often have difficulty with which of the following school related tasks?

    A. Drawing, building with blocks, and assembling a science model.
    B. Meeting physical education requirements, cutting with scissors, and playing a musical instrument.
    C. Attending to tasks, remaining seated, and remembering verbal information.
    D. Reading, memorizing multiplication tables, and using a computer keyboard.

30. An OTR has received a referral from a nursing home requesting adaptive self-care equipment for a patient with a C_5 spinal cord injury. The equipment that this patient would most likely be able to use independently is:

    A. shower chair.
    B. universal cuff.
    C. sliding board.
    D. sock aid.

31. An 8-year-old with developmental delay, who has learned to hold scissors correctly and to open and close them, is now ready to cut:

    A. a circle.
    B. random snips.
    C. along a line.
    D. a triangle.

32. After several weeks of treatment to achieve independence in self-care, a patient's endurance continues to be limited. The patient is barely able to complete self-care tasks before becoming completely fatigued. The patient's discharge date is ten days away. The patient wants to participate in his family's tradition of "family game night" which involves board games. The family indicates that they are willing to assist with his care in order for participation to occur. The OTR should:

    A. explain to the patient and family that the initially established goals must be met before adding additional goals.
    B. ask the patient and family to discontinue their tradition of "family game night" until the patient is stronger.
    C. alter the treatment plan to include the patient and family's goal to participate in "family game night."
    D. discourage the family from considering assisting with the patient's care.

33. A 79-year-old man who is obese has been admitted to the hospital with a hip fracture. He is restricted to touch down weight bearing for six weeks. The OTR observes that the patient does not recall his hip precautions and refuses to perform any self-care tasks. After consulting with the patient and his 79-year-old wife, which of the following settings would provide the most appropriate placement for this patient?

    A. At home with home health therapy services only.
    B. At home with an exercise program and care by his wife.
    C. A retirement home for the remainder of the six weeks.
    D. A skilled nursing facility with therapy services for six weeks.

34. An outpatient is referred by a physician for an OT evaluation. The patient's insurance company does not cover outpatient OT services. The therapist should:

    A. follow the physician's order and let the patient worry about the bill when it is received.
    B. provide the evaluation to the patient without charging for the service.
    C. explain the limitations of insurance coverage and let the patient decide whether to pursue the evaluation.
    D. request that the hospital billing department submit a bill using a code that is covered by the insurance company.

35. When preparing an OT program for a patient with multiple sclerosis, the program should include all of the following **EXCEPT**:

    A. gentle stretching of tight muscles.
    B. graded resistive exercises.
    C. very warm water exercises.
    D. energy conservation techniques.

36. The OTR learns that the home program recommended for a 6-year-old with spina bifida is not being carried out. In this situation, the therapist should **FIRST**:

    A. discontinue the home program and allow the caregiver to observe and participate during therapy sessions.
    B. reevaluate whether the home program corresponds with the understanding, the physical abilities, and the motivations of the caregiver.
    C. call a meeting for the purpose of impressing upon the caregiver the importance of follow-through at home.
    D. provide further instruction and demonstration of the home program activities during the next therapy session.

37. Participation in which of the following activities is **MOST** appropriate for an agitated patient who has auditory hallucinations and a short attention span?

A. Music group.
B. Task group.
C. Problem-solving group.
D. Discussion group.

38. An ambulatory elderly man with a primary diagnosis of middle-stage Alzheimer's disease is to be discharged home with his wife as caregiver. It is **MOST IMPORTANT** for the OT home program to contain:

A. methods to reduce environmental stimulation.
B. a reminder book to compensate for reduced memory.
C. memory enhancing cognitive exercises.
D. adaptive self-care equipment.

39. A patient is being treated by OT following a recent hip fracture and has been newly diagnosed with lung cancer. After initial progress in therapy, the patient has regressed. The patient is spending more and more time in bed, doing less self-care, and is not eating. The patient does not refuse therapy when offered; however, the patient does not actively participate in therapy. The OT program should be:

A. discontinued due to the inability to provide the plan as established.
B. revised in order to identify and prioritize the patient's goals.
C. continued according to the current plan with nonattendance documented.
D. increased in order to expand the patient's opportunity to participate.

40. A child experiencing tactile defensiveness:

A. lacks modulation of extraneous tactile input.
B. lacks hemispheric specialization.
C. has an overabundance of tactile receptors.
D. has decreased stereognosis skills.

41. OT documentation for each patient should contain all of the following information **EXCEPT:**

A. therapy intervention.
B. treatment techniques.
C. cost of treatment.
D. patient responses.

42. Quality assurance is critical in:

A. assessing service delivery.
B. accrediting schools.
C. certifying therapists.
D. reporting uniformly.

43. When patients who are on psychotropic medications are taken outdoors for activities in sunny weather, which of the following is **MOST** important for the OTR to instruct the patients to do?

A. Select indoor activities if they are sun sensitive.
B. Increase fluid intake before leaving and during the activities.
C. Obtain permission from their psychiatrists to discontinue medication for that day.
D. Wear a hat and sun block preparation on exposed areas of the skin.

44. If a child who is participating in a group of 6- to 8-year-olds with behavior problems becomes combative when frustrated, the OTR's **MOST APPROPRIATE** response would be to:

A. confront the aggressor.
B. institute a time-out system.
C. order the child to stop the behavior immediately.
D. discuss the behavior with the group.

45. Following the birth of her fifth child, a 25-year-old, unemployed female with an eighth grade education and diagnosis of depression and chronic substance abuse is referred to a day treatment center. The patient is despondent and has little belief in her ability to "stay off drugs." Her motivation appears to be very low. At this time, the **MOST** effective treatment activities would be those that:

A. provide concrete experiences in which the patient can obtain mastery and achievement.
B. focus on the effects that substance abuse has on the patient's health and quality of life.
C. expose the patient to the many opportunities that are available to her.
D. teach alternative coping mechanisms such as biofeedback and positive self-talk.

46. An OTR decides to use the principles of positive reinforcement with a patient who is repeatedly late for an activity group. The next time the patient is late, the OTR should:

A. advise the patient that this is inappropriate, and discuss with the patient what privileges will be lost if the behavior continues.
B. impress upon the patient the importance of being punctual to develop good work habits.
C. help the patient become aware of what emotions are being hidden by this passive aggressive behavior through expressive media.
D. disregard the tardiness and give a special reward to all who arrived on time.

47. A patient has been newly diagnosed with chronic obstructive pulmonary disease. The OTR receives a referral to prepare a home program. The OT home program should include all of the following **EXCEPT:**

A. utilization of pursed lip breathing techniques.
B. avoidance of items with strong odor.
C. lying flat when fatigued or short of breath.
D. participation in relaxation activities daily.

48. A patient with obsessive-compulsive personality disorder is being treated in an acute care psychiatric setting. The OTR is helping the family members understand the disorder and its effect on the patient's occupational functioning. From a psychodynamic orientation, the disorder is best explained as:

A. a need for recognition.
B. a need for achievement.
C. a need to control anxiety.
D. a need for immediate gratification.

49. An OTR works part-time at an inpatient treatment facility as well as being a self-employed contractor to several group homes. Is it the responsibility of the OTR to obtain individual malpractice and liability insurance for the contracted work?

A. Yes, it is the responsibility of an OTR working as an independent contractor to carry individual liability coverage.
B. No, liability insurance from the OTR's primary work setting provides comprehensive coverage.
C. No, it is the responsibility of the group homes to carry liability insurance for their contracted service providers.
D. Yes, liability coverage from the inpatient setting is nullified if the OTR takes on private clients.

50. An OTR receives a referral from a physician that outlines a specific course of treatment. Following the evaluation of the patient, the OTR believes that a different course of treatment would be more beneficial to the patient. The **BEST** course of action for the OTR is to:

A. give the prescribed treatment a three- or four-week trial.
B. contact the physician and suggest an alternative treatment.
C. combine the prescribed treatment with the treatment that the OTR believes to be more beneficial.
D. proceed with the treatment that the OTR believes would be more beneficial for the patient.

Answer Key for Study Guide OTR Test

1-B
2-C
3-C
4-D
5-A
6-D
7-B
8-B
9-B
10-A
11-A
12-D
13-A
14-A
15-A
16-D
17-A
18-B
19-B
20-A
21-B
22-C
23-C
24-B
25-D
26-C
27-A
28-B
29-A
30-B
31-B
32-C
33-D
34-C
35-C
36-B
37-B
38-A
39-B
40-A
41-C
42-A
43-D
44-B
45-A
46-D
47-C
48-C
49-A
50-B

3. Which of the following deficits may be present as a result of a peripheral nerve injury?

   A. Spasticity, decreased muscle strength, and decreased active ROM.
   B. Decreased passive ROM, impaired sensation, and tremor.
   C. Decreased active ROM, decreased muscle tone, and impaired coordination.
   D. Impaired motor planning, decreased muscle strength, and decreased active ROM.

   Correct Answer: C.
   C. Peripheral nerve injury causes a lack of innervation to specific muscles, resulting in deficits in active ROM, muscle tone, muscle strength, sensation, and coordination.

   A. This answer is incorrect because of the inclusion of spasticity. Spasticity occurs as a result of central nervous system lesion, and is not seen as a result of peripheral nerve injury.

   B. This answer is incorrect because of the inclusion of tremor. Tremor is generally seen following central nervous system damage, and is not a symptom of a peripheral nerve injury.

   D. This answer is incorrect because of the inclusion of motor planning. Motor planning is a central nervous system function, and is not impaired as a result of peripheral nerve injury.

4. An OTR observes another OTR using an incorrect technique to complete a stand pivot transfer with a patient. The OTR who observes the improper transfer has a responsibility to:

   A. report the matter to the OT supervisor immediately.
   B. report it to the OT supervisor if it happens again.
   C. instruct the therapist in the proper technique with the patient present.
   D. talk with the therapist in private about proper stand pivot transfer technique.

   Correct Answer: D.
   D. This approach represents a discreet and respectful intervention.

   A. A matter like this does not need to be reported unless the therapist continues to use the incorrect technique after instruction.

   B. This type of situation can not be ignored because a patient may be injured.

   C. This approach might interfere with the patient-therapist relationship.

5. A realistic functional goal for a patient with complete C_4 quadriplegia would be:

A. operation of a computer using a head switch.
B. independence in sliding board transfer.
C. independence in upper-extremity dressing.
D. self-feeding with wrist support and adaptive utensils.

Correct Answer: A.

A. A patient with complete C_4 quadriplegia has active shoulder elevation only, and is therefore dependent both on others and on adaptive equipment for almost all ADL activities. A head switch or sip and puff switch can be used for accessing a computer. This would be an important functional goal.

B. A patient with complete C_4 quadriplegia would be dependent for all transfers due to limited innervation in the shoulder girdle musculature and lack of trunk stability.

C. A patient with complete C_4 quadriplegia would need maximal assistance with all dressing activities.

D. A patient with complete C_4 quadriplegia might be able to perform self-feeding, but would require a fully powered orthosis to compensate for the lack of active elbow and shoulder flexion.

6. Which of the following approaches is **LEAST** threatening to an adolescent with schizophrenia who is withdrawn and apprehensive?

A. Allowing permissiveness.
B. Providing close supervision.
C. Providing a variety of activities.
D. Establishing a set schedule.

Correct Answer: D.

D. The establishment of a set schedule will provide this patient with a certain degree of predictability in daily routine, which will foster an increased sense of security in the environment.

A,C. Both of these options are too unstructured for a patient with schizophrenia who is withdrawn and apprehensive. These open-ended options are too unstructured for a patient with disorganized thought patterns.

B. Close supervision could be seen as invasive by this patient. Also, the therapist should take into account that this is an adolescent, an age where some degree of independence and choice are important factors to consider in treatment planning.

7. An OTR is performing a motor assessment on a child with cerebral palsy. When the child turns his head to look at an object placed in his hand, his arm extends and he drops the object. The OTR suspects that this is due to:

   A. poorly coordinated visual pursuits.
   B. asymmetrical tonic neck reflex.
   C. poorly integrated grasp reflex.
   D. upper extremity spasticity.

   Correct Answer: B.

   B. In the asymmetrical tonic neck reflex (ATNR), turning of the head results in extension of the upper extremity on the face side and flexion of the upper extremity on the skull side. Although the response of the skull side arm is not described here, the fact that the extension pattern of the face side arm occurs as a result of the head turning would lead the therapist to hypothesize that this is due to the influence of the ATNR.

   A. Although visual pursuits may be poorly coordinated in a child with cerebral palsy, they are not the cause of this particular response.

   C. If the grasp reflex had not been integrated, the child would not have been able to let go of the object.

   D. Although upper extremity spasticity may be present, it is the influence of the ATNR that causes the specific response described here.

8. A patient unable to "blow" on command can spontaneously blow out a match placed in front of the face. This is an example of which of the following deficits?

   A. Agnosia.
   B. Ideomotor apraxia.
   C. Ataxia.
   D. Constructional apraxia.

   Correct Answer: B.

   B. The inability to blow on command is an example of ideomotor apraxia. The patient is able to carry out an activity spontaneously but is unable to perform the task on verbal command.

   A. Agnosia is the inability to recognize familiar objects. This might be seen when a patient attempts to brush his/her teeth with a comb.

   C. Ataxia is an impairment of movement resulting from a brain lesion. This movement impairment results in a lack of coordination, unsteady gait, and poor balance.

   D. Constructional apraxia is the inability to produce designs whether two dimensional or three dimensional.

9. The Medicare program was designed **PRIMARILY** to provide medical coverage for:

A. low-income persons.
B. people aged 65 and over.
C. retired persons.
D. people who have been disabled for 12 months or more.

Correct Answer: B.
B. Medicare was enacted to provide medical coverage to persons 65 years of age and older.

A. Medicaid is the program that addresses the needs of persons with low-income under the age of 65 and is state administered.

C. Many retired persons may not be 65 years of age or older.

D. Medicare does provide some medical coverage for persons with specific disabling conditions; however, they have to have been receiving Social Security disability checks for 24 months before coverage begins.

10. Which of the following would be **MOST** difficult for a child with motor planning problems to perform on a scooter board?

A. Sitting on the scooter board and pulling self along a taut rope with hand-over-hand motion.
B. Maintaining prone position while being pushed through an obstacle course.
C. Maintaining balance on the scooter board while being pulled by the OTR.
D. Going down a ramp in prone position with legs extended.

Correct Answer: A.
A. This activity requires the child to plan and execute bilateral alternating movements while seated on the scooter board. Of the four activities listed, this would be the most difficult for a child with poor motor planning skills.

B,C,D. These three activities primarily require the child to maintain balance in a particular position on the scooter board while being moved. None of these activities require a significant amount of motor planning ability.

11. Which of the following statements is an example of objective data when writing a SOAP note?

   A. The patient has 30 degrees of elbow flexion.
   B. The patient will be able to achieve 50 degrees of elbow flexion.
   C. The patient is unable to comb hair due to arm pain.
   D. "I cannot move my right arm without it hurting."

   Correct Answer: A.
   A. This is an objective finding made by the therapist.

   B. This is a goal statement and belongs in the plan portion of the note.

   C. This is an assessment of how the pain limits the patient's functional ability.

   D. This belongs in the subjective part of the note because it is a statement made by the patient.

12. An OTR employed in a public school is asked to give a presentation to parents and staff regarding the role of OT in a special education program. Which of the following would be **MOST** effective in presenting the scope of educationally related OT services to this audience?

   A. A description of the types of assessments used to identify students in need of OT services.
   B. A demonstration of equipment most frequently used by school-based OTRs.
   C. A simulation of a therapy session with a child from the OTR's caseload.
   D. A discussion of problems typically addressed by school-based OTRs and service delivery options.

   Correct Answer: D.
   D. By discussing problems typically seen by OTRs, the audience will be able to get an idea of the breadth and scope of OT treatment in the schools. Discussion of service delivery options will further expand the audience's knowledge of the types of children seen for therapy and the levels and types of services available.

   A. This information would probably be too technical, and would not be of general interest for this audience.

   B. This might limit the audience's perception of OT in the schools to that of someone who works only with children who have severe motor impairments.

   C. This would also provide a narrow view of the role of the OT in schools.

13. An OTR observes that a patient with a spinal cord injury has an improperly fitting wheelchair. The **MOST IMMEDIATE** safety concern of the OTR would be the patient's:

    A. skin integrity.
    B. development of scoliosis.
    C. being unable to propel the wheelchair.
    D. being uncomfortable because of the height of the armrests.

    Correct Answer: A.

    A. Pressure sores can develop if too much pressure is exerted over bony prominences for too long.

    B. Scoliosis could be a long term concern but would not be the most immediate concern.

    C. The inability to propel the wheelchair would cause a functional problem but would not represent an immediate safety issue.

    D. While the position of the armrests is important to the overall positioning of the patient, it would not be the most immediate safety concern.

14. A patient is working on a copper tooling project and cuts his finger. The OTR should **FIRST:**

    A practice universal precautions and apply direct pressure to the wound.
    B. contact the physician before initiating any treatment.
    C. document the incident and have the patient return to his room.
    D. report the injury to the patient's nurse.

    Correct Answer: A.

    A. This is standard first aid procedure for a small cut and should be performed immediately.

    B. The physician may not need to be contacted if the cut is small. This would not be the first action.

    C. The injury needs to be documented; however, this can be done after the patient has been treated.

    D. The patient's nurse should be notified after the first aid is provided. The nurse is in charge of the patient's overall care and can follow up with necessary procedures and protocol.

15. How should paints and paint thinners be stored in an OT clinic?

    A. In a well-ventilated closed metal cabinet.
    B. On shelves in a locked storeroom.
    C. In a well-ventilated closed wooden cabinet.
    D. On open shelves in the craft area.

    Correct Answer: A.

    A. Paint and paint thinners are very flammable and should be stored in a well-ventilated closed metal cabinet. A metal cabinet provides a safe, noncombustible way to store flammable items.

    B. Paints and paint thinners stored on open shelves increases the chances of combustion.

    C. Flammable products should not be stored in a wooden cabinet because of the fire hazard.

    D. Storage on open shelves in the craft area is not safe due to the potential for exposure to sparks.

16. A 16-year-old adolescent who has a cognitive disability and an adjustment disorder, not otherwise specified, is being discharged to his family home from an acute care psychiatric setting. In planning for discharge, the **FIRST** activity for the OTR to consider would be:

    A. planning an appropriate home program.
    B. providing aftercare recommendations and referrals.
    C. educating the family and the patient for transition to community.
    D. evaluating the patient's home environment.

    Correct Answer: D.

    D. Because the patient has a cognitive disability, it is critical to assess the home environment first. This is the only way that safety issues and environmental concerns can be evaluated and addressed.

    A,B,C. These would all be important, but the home evaluation would be critical to the effectiveness of these other activities. As a general principle, evaluation would be done before planning.

17. An OTR receives a referral for a 12-month-old with spastic quadriplegic cerebral palsy. In addition to an assessment of motor development, which of the following types of evaluations are **MOST** appropriate in an initial assessment?

A. Reflex testing and feeding evaluation.
B. Reflex testing and sensory evaluation.
C. Visual perception evaluation and ADL evaluation.
D. Sensory evaluation and ADL evaluation.

Correct Answer: A.

A. Reflex testing is done to determine what primitive and/or abnormal reflexes are present and how they impact functional motor skills. A feeding evaluation is appropriate because of the strong possibility of oral involvement in a child with spastic quadriplegia.

B. Sensation may be evaluated in a 12-month-old but it is difficult to accurately assess at this age.

C. Visual perception may be evaluated in a 12-month-old but it is difficult to accurately assess at this age. It would generally not be part of the initial assessment. ADL assessment is not appropriate for a 12-month-old.

D. See answers B. and C.

QUESTIONS 18 AND 19 REFER TO THE FOLLOWING INFORMATION:

An 18-year-old female was hospitalized because she was unable to concentrate and unable to sleep. On admission, her speech was rapid, she was hyperactive, and she began organizing patients' activities for the evening. She became interested in several projects after entering OT.

18. Which of the following would be the **MOST APPROPRIATE** goal for this patient?

A. Improve work skills.
B. Increase self-control.
C. Increase frustration tolerance.
D. Increase problem-solving ability.

Correct Answer: B.

B. Increased self control is the first step before the patient will be able to address the other goals mentioned.

A,C,D. While these may be important goals for this patient after she gains more self control, they would not be appropriate at this time.

19. Which of the following would be the **MOST APPROPRIATE** activity for this patient to achieve the initial goal?

 A. Sketching.
 B. Tile project.
 C. Menu planning.
 D. Leather carving.

 Correct Answer: B.

 B. This is a structured activity which will enable the patient to increase her self-control.

 A,C. These are open ended activities and would not provide the structure needed by this patient.

 D. Since this patient is exhibiting decreased self-control, leather carving would be inappropriate due to the potential danger because of the use of sharp instruments.

20. A patient with spinal cord injury has difficulty dealing with anger about his limitations. Which of the following actions is an example of **projection** used as a defense mechanism?

 A. The patient tells the OTR that "50% of the nurses on the unit should be doing something else for a living. They think we're second class citizens just because we're in wheelchairs."
 B. During training in electric wheelchair skills, the patient frequently comments, "I can't wait to start riding my motorcycle again!"
 C. The patient tells the other patients that he is going to get his hair cut just like his therapist's and buy the same type of clothes as his therapist's.
 D. The patient states "I am going to get much better seats at the ball game now that I am in a wheelchair."

 Correct Answer: A.

 A. This is an example of the defense mechanism projection. Projection is the act of shifting responsibility for a feeling to another person instead of oneself.

 B. This is an example of the defense mechanism denial. Denial is a refusal to believe in reality to reduce its impact.

 C. This is an example of the defense mechanism identification. Identification is overvaluing someone more than his or her personality seems to merit.

 D. This is an example of the defense mechanism rationalization. Rationalization is finding an advantage to an undesirable situation.

21. Which of the following OT treatments is **NOT** recommended for patients with degenerative diseases of the central nervous system?

A. Instruction in energy conservation and work simplification techniques.
B. Establishment of an aggressive, resistive exercise program.
C. Provision of assistive devices.
D. Recommendation of workplace modifications.

Correct Answer: B.

B. While strengthening can be an appropriate goal, most degenerative diseases have inherent precautions against fatigue. The word aggressive in this answer raises questions about whether or not this precaution is being heeded.

A,C,D. These answers do not raise questions about precautions, and are appropriate treatment approaches for individuals with degenerative disease.

22. An 82-year-old who lives alone is forgetful, confused, and disoriented to time. Which of the following approaches would be **MOST** appropriate in assessing the self-care skills of this patient?

A. Interview the family regarding the patient's self-care skills.
B. Ask the patient to describe self-care routine.
C. Observe the patient's performance of self-care.
D. Interview the family regarding environmental safety hazards in patient's home.

Correct Answer: C.

C. Observation is the most direct method of assessing functional ability especially when the symptoms that are described are evident.

A. Interviews would provide valuable information but would not provide the most direct information regarding self-care skills. Also, the family may not have an accurate picture of the patient's skills.

B. This patient is forgetful, confused, and disoriented. It is unlikely that the reported information will be reliable.

D. The family may not be aware of environmental safety hazards in the house.

23. The length of time a child is able to attend to a task is most directly related to:

A. memory.
B. previous experience.
C. developmental age.
D. role expectations.

Correct Answer: C.

C. A child's attention span increases as a function of developmental age. If you had two children, one functioning at the five-year level and one functioning at the two-year level, you would not expect the child functioning at the two-year level to have an attention span as long as the child functioning at the five-year level.

A. Memory of the task may play a role in the child's interest in a task, but does not directly affect the child's attention span.

B. Previous experience is similar to memory. It may affect the child's interest and motivation in the task, which can affect attention span, but it does not directly relate to attention span.

D. Role expectations may impact attention span by affecting the child's perceptions of what is expected and therefore influence motivation for the task, but does not affect the child's cognitive ability to attend to that which is directly related to developmental age.

24. A 20-year-old patient hospitalized with a diagnosis of schizophrenia begins to hear voices and walks to the staircase to peer over. The patient says, "I want to kill the voices." The **MOST APPROPRIATE** response for the OTR would be to:

A. ask the patient to identify the voices.
B. talk to the patient while moving the patient from the staircase.
C. discuss the voices and why the patient wants to kill them.
D. tell the patient that the voices are not really there.

Correct Answer: B.

B. By talking with the patient, the therapist is acknowledging the patient's behavior and thought processes, while at the same time, ensuring increased safety for the patient.

A,C. By only addressing the voices issue, the therapist has not taken the necessary precautions to increase safety in the environment such as moving the patient away from the staircase.

D. Auditory hallucinations are often associated with delusional thought patterns which are fixed beliefs that cannot be changed. Telling the patient that the voices are not there has little therapeutic impact, and once again, does not address the safety issues.

25. Which of the following is the primary role of the OTR during the beginning phase of cardiac rehabilitation?

A. Assessment of vital signs during simulated work task evaluation.
B. Assessment of cardiovascular responses to sustained standing.
C. Initiation of a progressive upper extremity exercise program.
D. Identification of ways to decrease energy expenditure during self-care tasks.

Correct Answer: D.

D. During the initial phase, the patient is involved in a course of progressive, low-energy expenditure hospital activity. Adaptive aids and techniques are often necessary. Continued participation in ADL gives the patient a sense of control and independence.

A,B,C. These activities are too aggressive and would typically take place during later phases.

26. Which of the following would be a long-term goal for an adult with a sudden onset of blindness?

A. Independent coin identification and check writing.
B. Independent bathing, grooming, and dressing.
C. Independent living and exploration of employment options.
D. Independent time-telling and schedule management.

Correct Answer: C.

C. This goal is an example of a long-term goal. Long-term goals specify the end product of therapy. To achieve long-term goals, the therapist plans a series of short-term goals that lead to one or more long-term goals.

A,B,D. These can be seen as short-term goals leading to the long-term goal of independent living.

27. Mobile arm supports would help a person with proximal upper extremity weakness perform all of the following activities **EXCEPT:**

    A. upper body dressing.
    B. self-feeding.
    C. participation in tabletop board games.
    D. operation of an electric wheelchair.

    Correct Answer: A.
    A. Dressing requires more motion and more freedom of movement than is provided by mobile arm supports.

    B,C,D. These are all appropriate uses or training activities for individuals using mobile arm supports.

28. Which of the following activities would be **BEST** for assessing a patient's organizational and planning skills?

    A. Adding up the total coupon savings from a grocery bill.
    B. Preparing a grocery list for bag lunches for a group lunch.
    C. Studying home safety and listing the steps to put out a fire.
    D. Identifying the times for three programs using a TV schedule.

    Correct Answer: B.
    B. From the options presented, only this activity involves components of planning and organizing. The individual must plan what to put into the bag lunches then organize a list of items from the plan to compose the list, keeping in mind the size and needs of the group.

    A,C,D. These options require no planning or organizing, but rather adding, listing, and reading.

29. A child with constructional dyspraxia will often have difficulty with which of the following school-related tasks?

A. Drawing, building with blocks, and assembling a science model.
B. Meeting physical education requirements, cutting with scissors, and playing a musical instrument.
C. Attending to tasks, remaining seated, and remembering verbal information.
D. Reading, memorizing multiplication tables, and using a computer keyboard.

Correct Answer: A.

A. These tasks all require the ability to assemble components to make a whole. This ability is impaired in constructional apraxia.

B. These tasks require motor planning and eye-hand coordination abilities.

C. These tasks require the ability to maintain attention to the activity at hand. Specific praxis skills are not required.

D. These tasks require visual memory and figure-ground perception. Specific praxis skills are not required.

30. An OTR has received a referral from a nursing home requesting adaptive self-care equipment for a patient with a C_5 spinal cord injury. The equipment that this patient would most likely be able to use independently is:

A. shower chair.
B. universal cuff.
C. sliding board.
D. sock aid.

Correct Answer: B.

B. A universal cuff would compensate for the limited hand function demonstrated by individuals with C_5 spinal cord injury, and could be put on independently.

A,C,D. These pieces of adaptive equipment could not be used independently by a patient with a C_5 spinal cord injury.

31. An 8-year-old with developmental delay, who has learned to hold scissors correctly and to open and close them, is now ready to cut:

A. a circle.
B. random snips.
C. along a line.
D. a triangle.

Correct Answer: B.
B. A child just beginning to use scissors is not developmentally ready to cut specific lines. In the developmental sequence of scissor skills, random snips would be the next appropriate task.

A,C,D. The sequence of scissor skills from easiest to hardest would be snips, line, triangle, and then circle.

32. After several weeks of treatment to achieve independence in self-care, a patient's endurance continues to be limited. The patient is barely able to complete self-care tasks before becoming completely fatigued. The patient's discharge date is ten days away. The patient wants to participate in his family's tradition of "family game night" which involves board games. The family indicates that they are willing to assist with his care in order for participation to occur. The OTR should:

A. explain to the patient and family that the initially established goals must be met before adding additional goals.
B. ask the patient and family to discontinue their tradition of "family game night" until the patient is stronger.
C. alter the treatment plan to include the patient and family's goal to participate in "family game night."
D. discourage the family from assisting with the patient's care.

Correct Answer: C.
C. Collaboration with the family and or patient is an important part of all treatment planning. At times, assisting with the patient's care thereby allowing the patient to participate in meaningful activities is very important.

A. Goals can and should be modified as necessary to integrate the patient back into his or her family role.

B. This disregards the family's wishes.

D. This approach does not take into account the patient's goal of participating in "family game night." This patient doesn't have sufficient endurance to meet his personal goal and complete self-care independently.

33. A 79-year-old man who is obese has been admitted to the hospital with a hip fracture. He is restricted to touch down weight bearing for six weeks. The OTR observes that the patient does not recall his hip precautions and refuses to perform any self-care tasks. After consulting with the patient and his 79-year-old wife, which of the following settings would provide the most appropriate placement for this patient?

A. At home with home health therapy services only.
B. At home with an exercise program and care by his wife.
C. A retirement home for the remainder of the six weeks.
D. A skilled nursing facility with therapy services for six weeks.

Correct Answer: D.

D. Placement options need to be considered based on functional level and additional need for therapy or medical interventions. Safety precautions and the abilities of caregivers should also be considered. A skilled nursing facility is the only option listed which can provide adequate care and safety for this individual.

A. The home health therapy services would not cover enough of the day to assure his safety and compliance with precautions.

B. The exercise program would not provide him with sufficient therapy to regain safe performance of ADL with adaptive equipment as needed.

C. He does not meet the level of independence required for a retirement home.

34. An outpatient is referred by a physician for an OT evaluation. The patient's insurance company does not cover outpatient OT services. The therapist should:

A. follow the physician's order and let the patient worry about the bill when it is received.
B. provide the evaluation to the patient without charging for the service.
C. explain the limitations of insurance coverage and let the patient decide whether to pursue the evaluation.
D. request that the hospital billing department submit a bill using a code that is covered by the insurance company.

Correct Answer: C.

C. The patient has a right to be informed of the cost of services and to make his or her own decision concerning the ability to pay for therapy.

A. Not advising the patient of potential costs would be inconsiderate and would potentially place the patient in a poor financial situation.

B. It is not the therapist's right to determine whether services should be provided free of charge.

D. This would be fraudulent billing which is unethical and illegal.

35. When preparing an OT program for a patient with multiple sclerosis, the program should include all of the following **EXCEPT**:

A. gentle stretching of tight muscles.
B. graded resistive exercises.
C. very warm water exercises.
D. energy conservation techniques.

Correct Answer: C.

C. Heat can exacerbate the symptoms of multiple sclerosis.

A. Gentle stretching is appropriate to prevent contractures.

B. Carefully monitored resistive exercise is useful for increasing strength and physical conditioning.

D. Energy conservation techniques are important to decrease excessive fatigue.

36. The OTR learns that the home program recommended for a 6-year-old with spina bifida is not being carried out. In this situation, the therapist should **FIRST**:

A. discontinue the home program and allow the caregiver to observe and participate during therapy sessions.

B. reevaluate whether the home program corresponds with the understanding, the physical abilities, and the motivations of the caregiver.

C. call a meeting for the purpose of impressing upon the caregiver the importance of follow-through at home.

D. provide further instruction and demonstration of the home program activities during the next therapy session.

Correct Answer: B.

B. The caregiver needs to be involved in the home program from the beginning. The caregiver has the control over the home program; therefore, the home program must be accepted by the caregiver.

A. To discontinue the home program without evaluating what is going on at home would not provide the best solution to this situation. Just because the caregiver participates in the therapy session does not mean that the recommended activities will be done at home.

C. This could be a third step after reevaluating the home program and demonstrating the home program again.

D. This would be the second step after reevaluating the home program with the caregiver. If the caregiver does not understand the home program, instruction and demonstration may be helpful.

37. Participation in which of the following activities is **MOST** appropriate for an agitated patient who has auditory hallucinations and a short attention span?

    A. Music group.
    B. Task group.
    C. Problem-solving group.
    D. Discussion group.

    Correct Answer: B.
    B. A task group meets to create a product other than a meal. Involvement in such a group attempts to refocus the patient's attention from the hallucinations to a more structured task.

    A. Since this patient is hallucinating, involvement in a music group may not create enough structure for this patient and may also overstimulate this patient.

    C. Group problem solving is a higher level function and requires more sophisticated interpersonal communication skills than this patient is exhibiting.

    D. A discussion group might only encourage the patient to verbalize his hallucinations; thus, this patient is not exhibiting the appropriate behavior for such a group.

38. An ambulatory elderly individual with a primary diagnosis of middle-stage Alzheimer's disease is to be discharged home with a caregiver. It is **MOST IMPORTANT** for the OT home program to contain:

    A. methods to reduce environmental stimulation.
    B. a reminder book to compensate for reduced memory.
    C. memory enhancing cognitive exercises.
    D. adaptive self-care equipment.

    Correct Answer: A.
    A. For safety purposes at this stage of the disease, it is important to reduce the amount of stimulation to which the patient has to respond.

    B. At this stage, memory is not sufficient to use a reminder book.

    C. At any stage, memory is not expected to improve even with remediation.

    D. Most patients with middle-stage Alzheimer's disease are not able to comprehend the use of adaptive equipment.

39. A patient is being treated by OT following a recent hip fracture and has been newly diagnosed with lung cancer. After initial progress in therapy, the patient has regressed. The patient is spending more and more time in bed, doing less self-care, and is not eating. The patient does not refuse therapy when offered; however, the patient does not actively participate in therapy. The OT program should be:

A. discontinued due to the inability to provide the plan as established.
B. revised in order to identify and prioritize the patient's goals.
C. continued according to the current plan with non-attendance documented.
D. increased in order to expand the patient's opportunity to participate.

Correct Answer: B.
B. OT protocol for the treatment of individuals with cancer calls for optimizing function and considering the patient's goals in treatment planning.

A. A plan should not be discontinued without an attempt at revision, taking into account complicating factors.

C. The current plan has been demonstrated to be ineffective. Proceeding without modifying the treatment plan would be nonproductive.

D. Increasing the amount of OT does not necessarily increase the patient's participation.

40. A child experiencing tactile defensiveness:

A. lacks modulation of extraneous tactile input.
B. lacks hemispheric specialization.
C. has an overabundance of tactile receptors.
D. has decreased stereognosis skills.

Correct Answer: A.
A. Tactile defensiveness is defined as a disorder of the modulation or regulation of tactile sensory input.

B. Tactile processing does not take place at the hemispheric level, so lack of hemispheric specialization does not contribute to tactile defensiveness.

C. Children with tactile defensiveness have the same number of tactile receptors as other children. The difficulty lies in the child's ability to process the information that comes into the central nervous system through the receptors.

D. Stereognosis is a form of tactile discrimination. Tactile discrimination disorders are a separate condition from tactile defensiveness.

41. OT documentation for each patient should contain all of the following information **EXCEPT:**

A. therapy intervention.
B. treatment techniques.
C. cost of treatment.
D. patient responses.

Correct Answer: C.
C. The actual OT documentation need not include information regarding the cost of services.

A,B,D. Competent documentation of these aspects of treatment will facilitate the therapist's recall of treatment information and may assist the treatment team in treating the patient. These are also the aspects of the record which may be used for legal purposes.

42. Quality assurance is critical in:

A. assessing service delivery.
B. accrediting schools.
C. certifying therapists.
D. reporting uniformly.

Correct Answer: A.
A. By definition, the purpose of quality assurance is to provide a tool for assessing service delivery.

B,C,D. These are aspects of quality. An inspection of quality would certainly be a part of accrediting schools, certification of therapists, and uniform reporting; however, the term quality assurance is not used in these situations.

43. When patients on psychotropic drugs are taken outdoors for activities in sunny weather, which of the following is **MOST** important for the OTR to instruct the patients to do?

A. Select indoor activities if they are sun sensitive.
B. Increase fluid intake before leaving and during the activities.
C. Obtain permission from their psychiatrists to discontinue medication for that day.
D. Wear a hat and sun block preparation on exposed areas of the skin.

Correct Answer: D.

D. Various psychotropic drugs present the potential side effect of hypersensitivity to sunlight. To avoid skin irritation, it is recommended that a hat be worn and sun block be applied to exposed areas.

A. Excluding patients from an outing solely on the basis of sun sensitivity would be an over reaction by the therapist. Also, if excluded from the outing, these patients would not be learning how to cope with the side effects of the medication.

B. Although increasing fluid intake is a factor to consider when engaging in outdoor activities, this is not the most important issue.

C. The discontinuation of medication would be an inappropriate request by the therapist. This could have far-reaching implications on the patient's mental health status.

44. If a child who is participating in a group of 6- to 8-year-olds with behavior problems becomes combative when frustrated, the OTR's **MOST APPROPRIATE** response would be to:

A. confront the aggressor.
B. institute a time-out system.
C. order the child to stop the behavior immediately.
D. discuss the behavior with the group.

Correct Answer: B.

B. A time-out system provides a consistent method of discipline to be provided by the therapist. The time-out removes the child from the group, which decreases the likelihood of reinforcement for combative behavior. Behavior that is not reinforced is less likely to be repeated in the future.

A,C,D. These three actions provide reinforcement to the aggressor. If this combative behavior is reinforced, it could increase frequency and/or encourage other group members to demonstrate such behavior.

45. Following the birth of her fifth child, a 25-year-old, unemployed female with an eighth grade education and diagnosis of depression and chronic substance abuse is referred to a day treatment center. The patient is despondent and has little belief in her ability to "stay off drugs." Her motivation appears to be very low. At this time, the **MOST** effective treatment activities would be those that:

A. provide concrete experiences in which the patient can obtain mastery and achievement.
B. focus on the effects that substance abuse has on the patient's health and quality of life.
C. expose the patient to the many opportunities that are available to her.
D. teach alternative coping mechanisms such as biofeedback and positive self-talk.

Correct Answer: A.

A. These experiences are integral to instilling the belief in self necessary to overcome dependency.

B. Because of this patient's history she has probably had exposure to substance abuse education previously.

C. This patient's low motivation will impede any efforts to introduce her to new opportunities.

D. Alternative coping mechanisms may be useful later, but are premature until a foundation of motivation and a sense of competency are established.

46. An OTR decides to use the principles of positive reinforcement with a patient who is repeatedly late for an activity group. The next time the patient is late, the OTR should:

A. advise the patient that this is inappropriate, and discuss with the patient what privileges will be lost if the behavior continues.
B. impress upon the patient the importance of being punctual to develop good work habits.
C. help the patient become aware of what emotions are being hidden by this passive aggressive behavior through expressive media.
D. disregard the tardiness and give a special reward to all who arrived on time.

Correct Answer: D.

D. Based on the principles of positive reinforcement, the OTR would not respond to the tardiness. Addressing the tardiness would reinforce it and therefore increase the frequency this behavior.

A. This action is punishment and incongruent with positive reinforcement principles.

B. This is not an example of positive reinforcement because attention is being given to the negative behavior.

C. This action would only be appropriate if practicing from a psychodynamic orientation.

47. A patient has been newly diagnosed with chronic obstructive pulmonary disease. The OTR receives a referral to prepare a home program. The OT home program should include all of the following **EXCEPT:**

A. utilization of pursed lip breathing techniques.
B. avoidance of items with strong odor.
C. lying flat when fatigued or short of breath.
D. participation in relaxation activities daily.

Correct Answer: C.

C. Lying flat does not allow for proper drainage of secretions and can increase coughing or shortness of breath.

A. This technique is often recommended because it maintains a proper level of oxygen saturation.

B. Strong odors are known to exacerbate symptoms of chronic obstructive pulmonary disease.

D. These are used to help with sleeping and coping with panic attacks.

48. A patient with obsessive-compulsive personality disorder is being treated in an acute care psychiatric setting. The OTR is helping the family members understand the disorder and its effect on the patient's occupational functioning. From a psychodynamic orientation, the disorder is best explained as:

A. a need for recognition.
B. a need for achievement.
C. a need to control anxiety.
D. a need for immediate gratification.

Correct Answer: C.

C. Obsessive-compulsive personality disorder functions to control anxiety. It allows the patient to avoid the thoughts that arouse anxiety by focusing on external behaviors which must be performed.

A. Though society often confuses perfectionism with this disorder, the behaviors manifested by this type of patient will not be those that would accrue recognition of others.

B. The patient with obsessive-compulsive personality disorder experiences no accomplishment as a result of this disorder, the observed behaviors are never-ending and offer no sense of completion.

D. Obsessive-compulsive personality disorder offers the patient little opportunity for even minimal gratification due to its repetitive nature.

49. An OTR works part-time at an inpatient treatment facility as well as being a self-employed contractor to several group homes. Is it the responsibility of the OTR to obtain individual malpractice and liability insurance for the contracted work?

A. Yes, it is the responsibility of an OTR working as an independent contractor to carry individual liability coverage.
B. No, liability insurance from the OTR's primary work setting provides comprehensive coverage.
C. No, it is the responsibility of the group homes to carry liability insurance for their contracted service providers.
D. Yes, liability coverage from the inpatient setting is nullified if the OTR takes on private clients.

Correct Answer: A.

A. Liability coverage for an OTR working in any kind of treatment facility extends only to the patients/clients treated under the auspices of that facility.

B,C. If an OTR works as a private contractor, it is the OTR's responsibility to obtain individual liability coverage for the patients/clients treated.

D. If an OTR treats private patients in addition to those treated at the inpatient facility, the malpractice and liability insurance of the inpatient facility is not affected.

50. An OTR receives a referral from a physician that outlines a specific course of treatment. Following the evaluation of the patient, the OTR believes that a different course of treatment would be more beneficial to the patient. The **BEST** course of action for the OTR is to:

A. give the prescribed treatment a three- or four-week trial.
B. contact the physician and suggest an alternative treatment.
C. combine the prescribed treatment with the treatment that the OTR believes to be more beneficial.
D. proceed with the treatment that the OTR believes would be more beneficial for the patient.

Correct Answer: B.

B. Anytime the OTR would like to change a prescribed treatment the referring physician must be contacted. Also, many insurers only pay for the prescribed treatment.

A. To provide the prescribed treatment when it is not the most beneficial treatment could be detrimental to the patient's progress.

C. If the therapist does not believe that the prescribed treatment will be beneficial to the patient, the therapist can not justify providing that treatment.

D. An OTR should not ignore a physician's referral for a prescribed treatment.

SECTION IV
Selected References

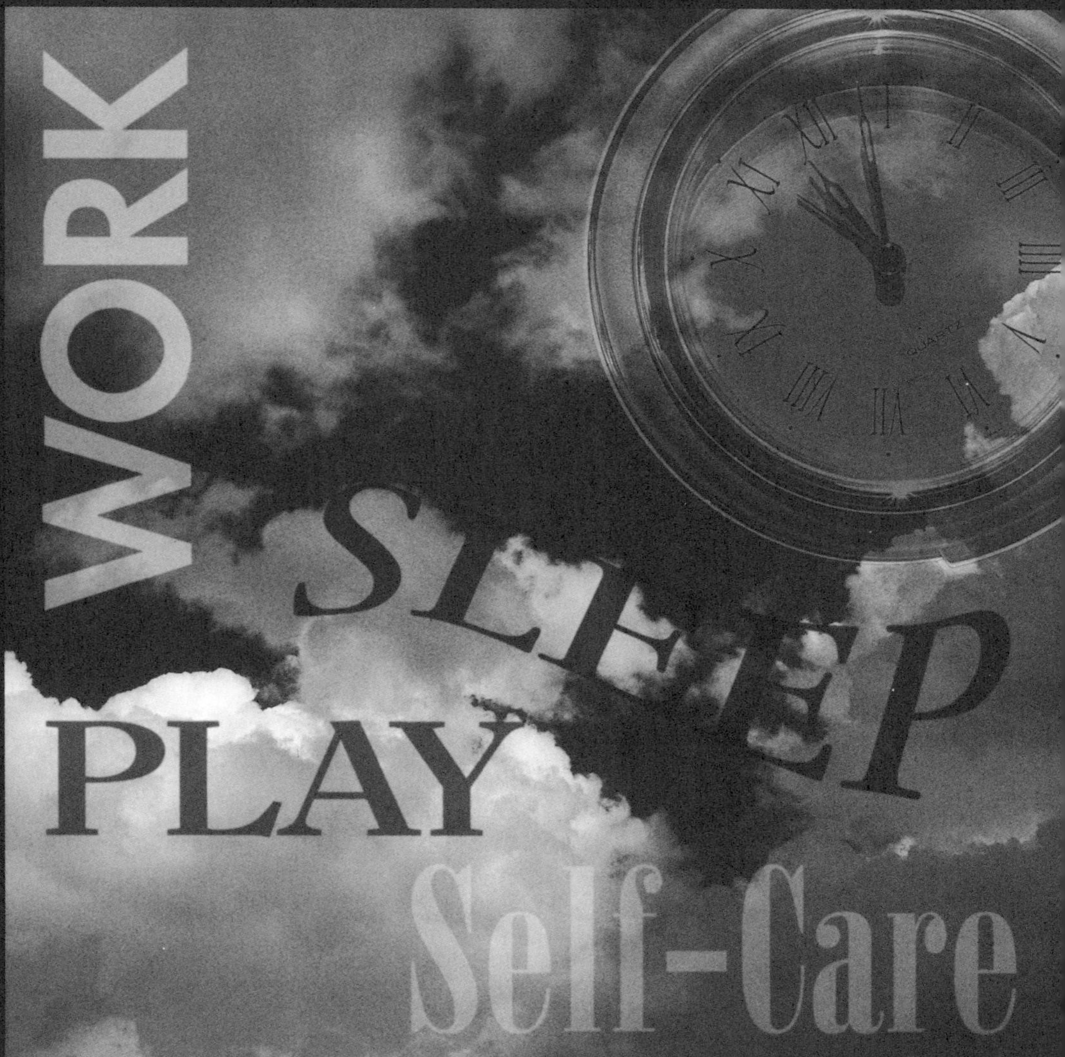

Selected References

The reference list below reflects the results of a survey of OTR program directors conducted in March 1993. The list represents the fourteen books most often recommended by the majority of the program directors for review by students taking the OTR certification examination.

It is recommended that candidates select their own reference sources based on previous coursework and areas of concentration in preparing for the examination. Where the candidate feels that he or she needs additional study, these reference materials may be helpful. **The provision of these references is not to be construed as an endorsement of these texts nor is it a guarantee that these are the only sources of references for the certification examination.**

Ayers, J. 1973. *Sensory Integration and Learning Disorders.* Western Psychological Services, Los Angeles, Ca.

Barris, R., G. Kielhofner, and J. Watts. *Bodies of Knowledge in Psychosocial Practice.* Slack, Inc, Thorofare, N.J.

Bruce, M. and B. Borg. 1993. *Frames of Reference in Psychosocial Occupational Therapy.* Slack, Inc., Thorofare, N.J.

Davis, L. and M. Kirkland. 1986. *The Role of OT with the Elderly.* AOTA, Rockville, Md.

Farber, S. 1982. *Neuro-Rehabilitation: A Multisensory Approach.* Saunders, Philadelphia, Pa.

Fiorentino, M. 1981. *A Basis for Sensorimotor Development: Normal and Abnormal: The Influence of Primitive, Postural Reflexes on the Development and Distribution of Tone.* Charles C. Thomas, Springfield, Ill.

Hemphill, B. 1988. *Mental Health Assessment in Occupational Therapy.* Slack, Inc, Thorofare, N.J.

Hopkins, H. and H. Smith. 1993. *Willard and Spackman's Occupational Therapy.* Lippencott, Philadelphia, Pa.

Howe, M. and S. Schwarztberg. 1986. *A Functional Approach to Group Work in OT.* Lippencott, Philadelphia, Pa.

Miller, B. R., et al. 1988. *Six Perspectives on Theory for the Practice of Occupational Therapy.* Aspen, Gaithersburg, Md.

Pedretti, L. 1990. *Occupational Therapy Practice Skills for Physical Dysfunction.* Mosby, St. Louis, Mo.

Pratt, P. and A. Allen. 1989. *Occupational Therapy for Children 2nd Edition.* Mosby, St. Louis, Mo.

Reed, K. and S. Nelson. 1992. *Concepts of Occupational Therapy.* Williams and Wilkins, Baltimore, Md.

Trombly, C. 1989. *Occupational Therapy for Physical Dysfunction.* Williams and Wilkins, Baltimore, Md.

Notes

Notes

Notes